INTERPRETING BASIC

CARDIAC DYSRHYTHMIAS

WITHOUT HEARTACHE

FIRST EDITION

Cheryl Miller, EdD, MSN, RN

PROFESSOR OF NURSING

Chattanooga State Community College

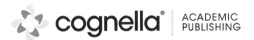

cognella® ACADEMIC PUBLISHING

Bassim Hamadeh, CEO and Publisher
Kassie Graves, Director of Acquisitions
Jamie Giganti, Senior Managing Editor
Jess Estrella, Senior Graphic Designer
Angela Schultz, Senior Field Acquisitions Editor
Michelle Piehl, Project Editor
Alexa Lucido, Licensing Coordinator
Berenice Quirino, Associate Production Editor

Printed in the United States of America

ISBN: 978-1-5165-0094-9 (pbk) / 978-1-5165-0095-6 (br)

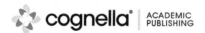

1-866-459

CONTENTS

INTRODUCTION

This book is about learning how to interpret basic electrocardiogram (EKG) readings. The author feels that by having a good understanding of normal sinus rhythm and the basic dysrhythmias, you can apply this knowledge and be able to understand and interpret the more advanced and difficult rhythms. Although it is not the primary purpose of the book, physiology and pathophysiology will be mentioned with each dysrhythmia to help promote a better understanding of what is happening within the heart. Again, even though it is not the intent of this book, common interventions/ medications will also be mentioned with each dysrhythmia. However, the reader should understand that this is not a comprehensive listing of all interventions and medications. The purpose of this book is for the reader to gain a greater understanding of how to interpret basic cardiac dysrhythmias. Also, this book is meant to pertain to adult clients, since rates and treatments may sometimes differ with children.

This book is divided into four sections. Practice strips with correct answers are provided in the fourth section.

Objectives

1. After reading Section I, one should be able to:

    1. Understand the conduction system of the heart

    2. Relate how an EKG works

    3. Interpret basic waveforms of an EKG reading

    4. Understand time as illustrated on an EKG reading

        i. Time and the PR interval

        ii. Time and the QRS complex

    5. Calculate atrial and ventricular rates

    6. Recognize normal sinus rhythm

    7. Apply a step-by-step process when interpreting strips

2. After reading Section II, one should be able to:

    1. Recognize common sinus dysrhythmias

        i. Understand basic physiology

        ii. State common interventions

    2. Interpret basic atrial dysrhythmias

        i. Understand basic physiology

        ii. State common interventions

3. After reading Section III, one should be able to:

    1. Identify atrioventricular heart blocks

        i. Understand basic physiology

        ii. State common interventions

    2. Recognize common ventricular dysrhythmias

        i. Understand basic physiology

        ii. State common interventions

3. Identify asystole

    i. Understand basic physiology

    ii. State common interventions

4. Understand the significance of pulseless electrical activity

4. In Section IV, one will be able to:

    1. Practice interpretation of the dysrhythmias discussed in Section II of this book

    2. Practice interpretation of the dysrhythmias discussed in Section III of this book

    3. Practice interpretation of all of the dysrhythmias in all sections of this book

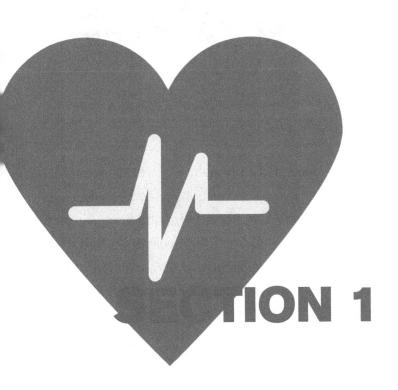

SECTION 1

Conduction System of the Heart

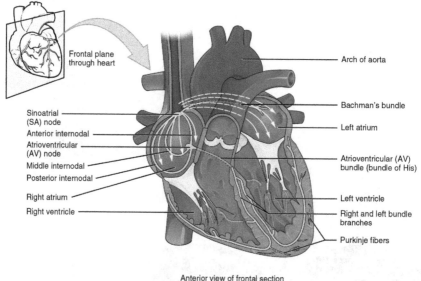

FIGURE 1-1. Conduction System of Heart

The very first thing you need to remember to begin interpreting cardiac dysrhythmias is the conduction system of the heart. Normally, the impulse for the heart to contract starts in the sinoatrial (SA) node. Then that impulse travels down through the internodal pathways to the atrioventricular (AV) node. The impulse is then transmitted to the bundle branches (right and left) and then finally ends in the Purkinje fibers.

The Electrocardiogram

All of the above activity is reflected on an EKG reading. Therefore, what an EKG reading represents is simply a measurement of the electrical activity or conduction occurring in the heart. If there is no electrical activity or conduction, the result is a straight line, which is also known as the baseline or isoelectric line. Any deviation from this isoelectric line shows that there is some type of electrical activity occurring. Let's look at this example.

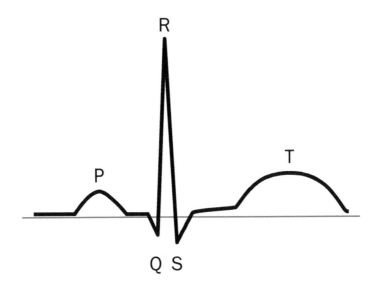

FIGURE 1-2. Isoelectric Line

Adapted from: Copyright © Mrug (CC BY-SA 3.0) at https://commons.wikimedia.org/wiki/
File%3ALinia_izoelektryczna_EKG.svg.

Can you identify the baseline or isoelectric line in the strip shown in Figure 1-2?

Waveforms on the EKG

Now look back at the above example in Figure 1-2. Notice the first deviation you see from the isoelectric line. Can you identify it? It is known as the P wave. What did you learn earlier about where the first impulse of the heart normally occurs? You are correct! It is in the SA node. When the SA node initiates an impulse and fires, the atria contract. This is what the P wave represents—contraction of the right and left atria.

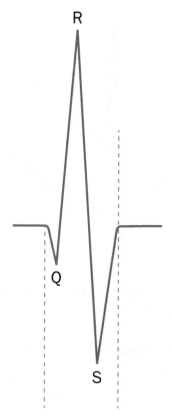

FIGURE 1-3. QRS Waveform

Adapted from: Copyright © Rob Kreuger (CC BY-SA 3.0) at https://commons.wikimedia.org/wiki/File%3AQRSwaves_(CardioNetworks_ECGpedia).jpg.

As the atria are contracting, the impulse is continuing to travel to the AV node. This event is known as the PR interval, and it is very important for you to calculate the time this takes. However, since you haven't learned how to measure time yet, just hold on to the following thought: As the atria are contracting, the impulse is continuing to the AV node, and the time required for this is known as the PR interval.

The next deviation from the isoelectric line that you should notice on the EKG strip shown above occurs after the P wave. It is a rather large and noticeable deviation, and it is known as the QRS complex. It is really three waves in one—the Q, the R, and the S. It is supposed to look something like the one illustrated in Figure 1-3.

Sometimes it may look different, and many times you may not even see the Q wave. However, it is still referred to as the QRS complex. It represents the next major activity of the heart, which is contraction of the ventricles. Since the ventricles are contracting, you know that the impulse has been received by the AV node and is traveling through the bundle branches and the Purkinje fibers as the ventricles contract.

It is important for you to know how long it is taking for the ventricles to contract. If it is taking longer than "normal," maybe there is a blockage of some type within the bundle branches or Purkinje fibers. Perhaps the impulse has not been traveling in a direct pathway from the AV node. Again, since you haven't learned about time on an EKG reading, just hold on to the following thought: The QRS complex should occur in a specified time and represents the time required for the ventricles to contract.

Now refer again to the EKG example illustrated in Figure 1-2. After the QRS complex, notice the next deviation from the isoelectric line. Can you find it?

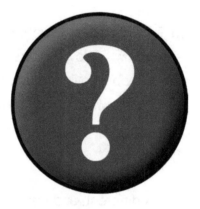

FIGURE 1-4. Question Mark

It is called the T wave. What do you think it represents? What else happens after the ventricles contract?

The T wave represents repolarization of the ventricles. What in the world does this mean?

Now is a good time for you to learn about three terms you need to understand. These terms are *polarization, depolarization,* and *repolarization.* Before an impulse is initiated, cardiac cells are in a resting phase or polarized phase. When an impulse reaches cardiac cells, it causes them to contract or depolarize. This involves a shift of electrolytes and ion charges across cell membranes, so it is denoted as activity and causes a deviation from the isoelectric line. Make a mental note of the fact that everything that depolarizes or contracts must repolarize. This is a return to the original resting or polarized state and also involves a shift of electrolytes and ions, so it causes a deviation from the isoelectric line on the EKG strip.

Therefore, the T wave represents repolarization of the ventricles. This has to occur for the ventricles ever to contract or depolarize again. **Everything that contracts or depolarizes has to repolarize!**

You need to practice a little thought exercise at this time. The question is: If everything that depolarizes has to repolarize, why didn't a waveform appear following atrial depolarization? Do they not have to repolarize?

What is your answer?

The answer is: *Yes, they do have to repolarize. You do not see a separate waveform because it is hidden when the ventricles contract. In other words, the QRS complex hides it. You know repolarization has to occur because without it the atria could not contract again.*

How did you do?

QUIZ # 1

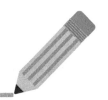

Let's review what you have learned so far. Take this little quiz to see how you are progressing.

1. What is the isoelectric line?

2. What does the P wave on an EKG reading represent?

3. What does the QRS complex on an EKG reading represent?

4. What does the T wave on an EKG reading represent?

5. What does the term *depolarization* mean?

6. What does the term *repolarization* mean?

QUIZ # 1 ANSWERS

1. It is the baseline on an EKG strip representing no electrical activity.

2. It represents contraction of the atria.

3. It represents contraction of the ventricles.

4. It represents repolarization of the ventricles.

5. *Depolarization* means contraction.

6. *Repolarization* means a return to the resting state, which makes the cell ready for another stimulus.

How did you do?

You have several more items to learn, so you'd better not take a break yet. It is very important that you completely understand the material you have just read. If you had trouble answering any of the questions in the above exercise, go back now and review before you continue.

Time Intervals

To understand the significance of each wave and interval, you now need to look at EKG paper and learn how time is measured on this paper. Notice in the example in Figure 1.5 that there are small and large blocks on the EKG paper. One small block represents 0.04 seconds on the horizontal line and 1 millivolt on the vertical line. Since a large block is five small blocks wide and five small blocks tall, each large block represent 0.20 seconds on the horizontal line and 5 millivolts on the vertical line. Notice that the horizontal line is the only one that deals with time. The vertical line deals with voltage or wattage, which will not be discussed as much since this is a book for basic interpretation of strips. For now you need to concentrate on just the horizontal line.

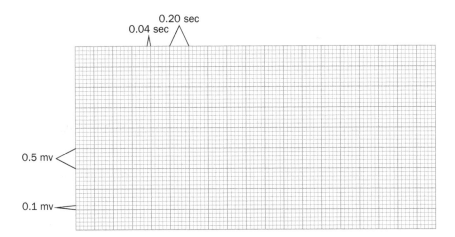

FIGURE 1-5. Time on EKG Paper

PR INTERVAL

Now you need to recognize the importance of knowing about the time element of EKG paper. Remember you learned earlier about the PR interval. Do you remember what it is and what it represents? Look at the example in Figure 1-6.

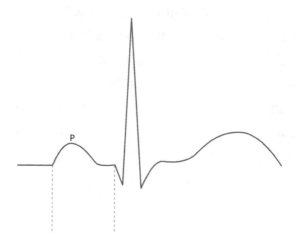

FIGURE 1-6. PR Interval Denoted by Dotted Lines

Copyright © Bran (CC BY-SA 3.0) at https://commons.wikimedia.org/wiki/File%3ANormal_PR_interval_(ECG).svg.

The PR interval extends from the beginning of the P wave to the onset of the Q wave. Wonder why it is call the PR interval instead of the PQ interval? Probably because many times you may not actually see a Q wave, but there will always be an R wave. Just look for the ending of the PR interval to be at the exact spot where the isoelectric line goes up or down before the QRS complex. Remember the PR interval represents conduction of the impulse throughout the atria and into the AV node. In normal situations the PR interval should be 0.12 to 0.20 seconds.

Think: How many small blocks is this?

Answer: Three to five small blocks, because remember each small block is 0.04 seconds.

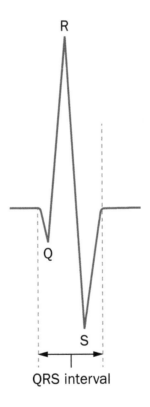

FIGURE 1-7. Measurement of the QRS Complex

QRS COMPLEX

Remember you also learned earlier how important it is for you to measure the QRS complex. This will allow you to know how long it is taking for the ventricles to contract. In normal situations the QRS complex should be 0.12 seconds or less. Therefore, this would be three small blocks or fewer on the EKG paper. The way the QRS interval is measured is demonstrated in Figure 1-7.

Calculating Rates

The time element of an EKG strip is also important when calculating the rate of a particular rhythm. When you take someone's pulse, aren't you calculating what the heart rate is for that person for 1 minute? Of course you are! Therefore, if you know what the heart rate is for 6 seconds on EKG paper, then you can predict what the rate will be for 60 seconds simply by multiplying by 10. Does this make sense?

Since you know that each horizontal big block is 0.20 seconds, if the EKG strip shows 30 big blocks, then you are looking at a 6-second strip (0.20 × 30 = 6 seconds).

So what does all of this mean? How can you calculate rate from all of this information?

Set your watch to go and try this next little quiz!

QUIZ # 2

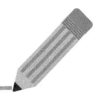

1. If you are trying to calculate the ventricular rate, what could you count on a 6-second strip and multiply by 10 to determine the rate for 1 minute?

2. If you are trying to calculate the atrial rate, what could you count on a 6-second strip and multiply by 10 to determine the rate for 1 minute?

QUIZ # 2 ANSWERS

1. The R waves

   Rationale: What represents contraction of the ventricles?
   The QRS complex does. However, since a Q wave may
   not always be present, the R wave is counted because it
   should always be present and is easy to locate.

2. The P waves

   Rationale: What represents contraction of the atria? The
   P waves do, of course!

   Well, how did you do?

   Try one additional quiz before you take a break.

QUIZ # 3

1. Determine the ventricular rate and the atrial rate on the two 6-second EKG strips in Figures 1-8 and 1-9.

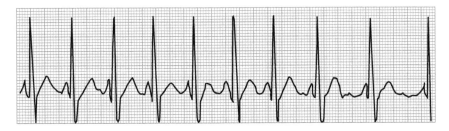

FIGURE 1-8.

What is the ventricular rate?

What is the atrial rate?

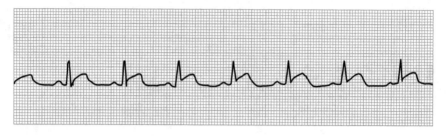

FIGURE 1-9.

What is the ventricular rate?

What is the atrial rate?

QUIZ # 3 ANSWERS

1. For Figure 1-8:

Ventricular rate: 100

Atrial rate: 100

For Figure 1-9:

Ventricular rate: 70

Atrial rate: 70

Well, how did you do? If you answered the questions in these two quizzes correctly, go have some lunch because you have almost mastered the basics of interpreting EKG strips. When you come back, you'll get into some real action!

If you are having trouble, go back and review one more time. You must understand all of this before you advance!

TAKE A BREAK!

Welcome back! Now's let's get you into some real action!

At this point you might be saying, "Hey, wait a minute. On the previous quiz, why did I have to determine the ventricular and atrial rates? Aren't they both always the same?"

Good point—but the answer is no!

In a normal healthy situation, they are usually the same, and this is an ideal situation. The best situation is for the atria to contract and fill the ventricles. Then the ventricles can contract and be full of blood, thereby giving a better cardiac output. They do this simultaneously, so the rates are the same.

However, there are many unhealthy situations where this does not occur. This is what the majority of the remainder of this packet will be about—these unhealthy situations where the impulse does not go as it should normally and where contraction does not occur as it should normally.

Before you continue, you need to review a few more important facts.

Pacing of the Heart

Think about the pacing that generally goes on in the heart. Remember the impulse is normally initiated in the SA node. The SA node normally discharges impulses at a rate of 60 to 100 times per minute. If for some reason the SA node fails to do this, the next normal pacemaker to take over would be the AV node. It can pace but usually at a slower rate of 40 to 60 times per minute. If for some reason the AV node fails, the Purkinje fibers can pace for a short while but at a much slower rate of 20 to 40 beats per minute. This is only temporary, however, and they won't be able to do this over a long period of time. This, however, is not the main problem when the Purkinje fibers are pacing. If the heart rate is 20 to 40, what do you think the cardiac output for that patient will be? You are correct! Not very good! Cardiac output is always the bottom line when you assess how your patient is doing. Remember these are general guidelines.

So that's simple enough—right?

Wrong!

Even though the conduction is expected to go through the SA, AV node, bundle of His, bundle branches, and Purkinje fibers, this is not always what occurs. Even though these tissues are specialized in the sense that they have automaticity and conductivity, they are not alone.

All myocardial cells have the ability to initiate an impulse under certain conditions! Many times, as you will see, they do just this!

As a general rule, the pacemaker firing at the fastest rate controls the heartbeat.

Also, to make things even more complicated, even though the SA node normally fires at 60 to 100 beats per minute, it can initiate higher or lower rates in some situations. For example, anxiety or a fever can cause the SA node to fire as high as 150 beats per minute. Usually it can go no higher than this. The AV node, in certain situations, can pace at higher or lower rates than its usual 40 to 60 beats per minute. The Purkinje fibers in the ventricles can do the same. Remember, though, you were told this is a basic beginner book. We are going to strive to keep your learning basic and simple so you can master this, and then more complicated dysrhythmias will be easy for you to interpret as you progress in your learning.

Wow, this is getting complicated!

Leads in Cardiac Monitoring

Next, you need to understand one more thing. You only will be working with strips that have been recorded in lead 2. This is a good thing! This is the easiest lead in which to interpret strips, and since this is a basic book, this is where you should begin. After you have mastered reading strips in lead 2, then you can begin to learn to read strips in other leads. These are usually taught in a critical-care course. So once again, all of your strips in this book will be in lead 2, and all strips will be 6-second strips.

Wait! You are not quite ready to begin yet. There's one more important piece of information you need to know before you launch into trying to interpret cardiac strips.

Step-by-Step Process in Interpreting Cardiac Strips

IMPORTANT: You will need to go through a step-by-step process in interpreting cardiac strips. If you omit one step, you may interpret incorrectly. Over time, this systematic approach will become second nature to you, but for now you need to go through each step.

These steps are as follows:

1. Scan the strip. Look for P waves, QRS complexes, and T waves. Look for any "odd" waveforms or premature beats—circle these if found.

2. Determine rates (atrial and ventricular).

3. State conduction ratio.

4. Determine rhythm.

5. Measure PR interval.

6. Measure QRS interval.

7. Identify dysrhythmia.

8. Identify source of impulse.

These will all be explained in greater detail when you read about normal sinus rhythm, which will be discussed next.

Mark these steps in your book because they hold the key to correctly interpreting dysrhythmias!

Also please note that the author of this book will use four steps in explaining all of the dysrhythmias that follow. They are:

1. The EKG strip will be shown.

2. A definition of the dysrhythmia on the strip will be given, along with basic physiology/pathophysiology. Some common causes may be mentioned.

3. The step-by-step process will be explained.

4. Basic interventions/treatments will be given at the end of each interpretation.

Let's get you started! You need to look at normal sinus rhythm first because this is a normal rhythm, not a dysrhythmia. A dysrhythmia is an abnormal rhythm. You will be comparing all dysrhythmias that follow to normal sinus rhythm to compare how they deviate. Make sense?

Let's go!

Normal Sinus Rhythm

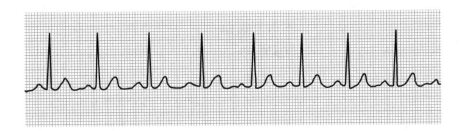

FIGURE 1-10. Normal Sinus Rhythm (NSR)

Definition: All beats appear in a similar pattern, are equally spaced, and have three major units: P wave, QRS complex, and T wave. Rate is normal—60 to 100 beats per minute. All time intervals (PR interval and QRS complex) are normal. Rhythm is regular.

 Interpreting the Strip

Step 1: Scan the strip: P waves, QRS complexes, and T waves are all present. There are no abnormal waveforms or premature waveforms.

Step 2: Rates: Ventricular rate is 80; atrial rate is 80. (The last P wave can be ignored since this is just where the next QRS is cut off in the strip). These both are within the normal SA node firing range of 60 to 100 beats per minute. P waves are present, and the PR interval is normal (see below), so the rate must be from the SA node.

Step 3: Conduction ratio: This is the number of QRS complexes for each P wave. You know this should be 1:1. This means that each time the atria contract, the ventricles contract, and the contractions are RELATED. In the above example, the conduction ratio is 1:1. You can determine this by scanning down the strip and seeing that there is a P wave before each QRS in the same order with each contraction. You also can simply note that the atrial and the ventricular rates are the same.

Step 4: Rhythm: To determine the ventricular rhythm, measure the distance between QRS complexes (Rs to Rs). For ventricular rhythm to be stated as regular, the QRS complexes should be the same distance apart. Sometimes a few may vary by one or two tiny, small squares, but basically you still should count that as regular. You will see what an irregular rhythm looks like later, and you can usually identify it very quickly. To determine the atrial rhythm, you should measure the distances between Ps, and they should be the same distance apart throughout the strip if the rhythm is regular. Determining rhythm is very important because you will soon be presented with dysrhythmias having irregular rhythms, so this will be a good clue for you. You will soon begin to realize that identifying a dysrhythmia on an EKG strip is much like working a crossword puzzle! In the example above, the atrial and ventricular rhythms are both regular. You can say that they each "march." There is the same distance between Ps (atrial rhythm) and between Rs (ventricular rhythm).

Step 5: PR interval: Remember you learned that the PR interval should be from 0.12 to 0.20 seconds (3 to 5 small blocks) when normal conduction is occurring between the SA and AV node. In the above strip, the PR interval is less than 0.20 seconds, so this is normal. Tip: Always look at all of the PR intervals to make sure they are the same.

Step 6: QRS complex: Also, remember you learned earlier that the QRS complex should be 0.12 seconds or less (3 small blocks or fewer) if conduction is occurring through the ventricles as it should. In the above strip, the QRS complex measures 0.04 seconds.

Step 7: Identify the rhythm: All the parameters appear to be normal, so your interpretation should be normal sinus rhythm. This is the rhythm that will be your model for "normal," and you will be comparing all other rhythms to this one.

Step 8: Determine the source of impulse: Since you have determined that the above rhythm is normal sinus rhythm, you know from your knowledge of physiology that the impulse for normal sinus rhythm is initiated by the SA node.

Interventions/Treatments

No interventions or treatments are indicated, since this is normal sinus rhythm.

Image Credits

- Fig. 1-1: Copyright © Openstax College (CC by 3.0) at https://commons. wikimedia.org/wiki/File%3A2018_Conduction_System_of_Heart.jpg.
- Fig. 1-2: Adapted from: Copyright © Mrug (CC BY-SA 3.0) at https:// commons.wikimedia.org/wiki/File%3ALinia_izoelektryczna_EKG.svg.
- Fig. 1-3: Adapted from: Copyright © Rob Kreuger (CC BY-SA 3.0) at https://commons.wikimedia.org/wiki/File%3AQRSwaves_(CardioNetworks_ECGpedia).jpg.
- Fig 1-4: Copyright © Tene~commonswiki (CC BY-SA 3.0) at https:// commons.wikimedia.org/wiki/File:Circle-question-red.svg#/media/ File:Circle-question-red.svg.
- Fig 1-6: Copyright © Bran (CC BY-SA 3.0) at https://commons.wikimedia.org/wiki/File%3ANormal_PR_interval_(ECG).svg.
- Fig 1-7: Copyright © Rob Kreuger (CC BY-SA 3.0) at https://commons. wikimedia.org/wiki/File%3AQRSwaves_(CardioNetworks_ECGpedia).jpg.

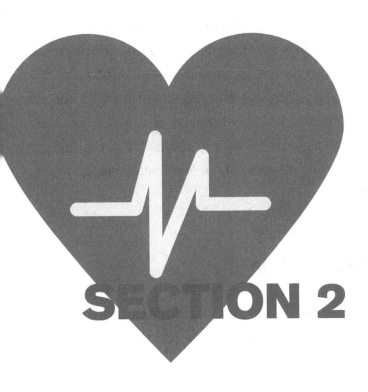

SECTION 2

Sinus Dysrhythmias

SINUS BRADYCARDIA

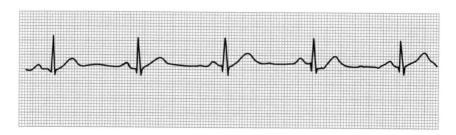

Figure 2-1. Sinus Bradycardia

Definition: All characteristics of normal sinus rhythm are present EXCEPT the rate. In sinus bradycardia the rate will be below 60 beats per minute. In this dysrhythmia the SA node is still firing, but something is causing it to fire slower than its normal pacing rate of 60 to 100 beats per minute. Some of the causes for this can be conditions such as hypothermia, digitalis toxicity, increased intracranial pressure, or vagal nerve stimulation (suctioning or gagging).

 ## Interpreting the Strip

Step 1: Scan the strip: P waves, QRS complexes, and T waves are all present. There are no abnormal or premature waveforms.

Step 2: Rates: The ventricular rate is 50, and the atrial rate is 50. Notice these are slower than normal sinus rhythm. This is your first deviation from normal sinus rhythm.

Step 3: Conduction ratio: 1:1. There is a P wave before each QRS complex, and they appear to be related. The P waves occur in the same place and always right before a QRS. This is showing that each time the atrial contract, the ventricles contract.

Step 4: Rhythm: The rhythm is regular. The Ps march (same distance apart), and the Rs march.

Step 5: PR interval: It is within normal limits—0.12 to 0.20 seconds (3 to 5 small blocks).

Step 6: QRS complex: It is within normal limits, which is 0.12 seconds or less (3 small blocks or fewer).

Step 7: Identify the dysrhythmia: Sinus bradycardia.

Step 8: Determine the source of impulse: Source of impulse is still the SA node. Remember it can pace at a slower rate under certain conditions, such as those listed above. You know that it is the SA node because there are P waves and the PR interval is normal.

Interventions/Treatments

The heart rate may need to be increased. It depends on how slow it is and if the client is symptomatic. A slow heart rate can cause decreased cardiac output, and this can cause the patient to be symptomatic. Do you remember what some signs of decreased cardiac output are? Yes, you are correct! Some of the signs and symptoms are decreased blood pressure, dizziness, fainting, and changes in orientation. The slower the heart rate becomes, the more likely signs and symptoms of decreased cardiac output will appear. Tip: A slightly slow heart rate is normal in some well-conditioned athletes because they have a larger stroke volume with each heartbeat, since cardiac muscle is well developed too! If this is the case, there will be NO signs of decreased cardiac output, so no treatment is necessary.

Probably the number one drug of choice to increase heart rate is atropine. Isoproterenol would also be an option.

SINUS TACHYCARDIA

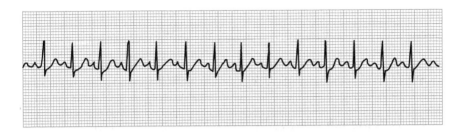

Figure 2-2. Sinus Tachycardia

Definition: All characteristics of normal sinus rhythm are present except the rate. In sinus tachycardia the atrial and ventricular rates will be 101 to 150 beats per minute. In this dysrhythmia the SA node is still firing the impulse, but something is causing it to fire at a faster rate than normal. Some conditions that can cause sinus tachycardia include fever, anxiety, stress, exercise, caffeine, and amphetamines.

 Interpreting the Strip

Step 1: Scan the strip: P waves, QRS waveforms, and T waves are all present. There are no abnormal waves or premature waves.

Step 2: Rates: The ventricular rate is 140, and the atrial rate is 140. Notice these are faster than normal sinus rhythm. This is your first deviation, so you know this is NOT normal sinus rhythm.

Step 3: Conduction ratio: 1:1

Step 4: Rhythm: Regular.

Step 5: PR interval: Within normal limits.

Step 6: QRS complex: Within normal limits.

Step 7: Identify the dysrhythmia: Sinus tachycardia.

Step 8: Determine the source of impulse: This is still the SA node. An important point to remember is that certain conditions, such as those listed above, can cause it to fire at a faster rate, but usually it cannot fire above 150 beats per minute.

 Interventions/Treatments

The heart rate needs to be slowed down. Cardiac output is compromised with a fast rate because the ventricles may not have adequate filling time. An increased rate also causes the heart to work harder and consume more oxygen; this is especially hard for patients whose hearts are already compromised, such as clients diagnosed with various heart conditions. Interventions are usually medications. These include drugs such as beta blockers, calcium channel blockers, and digitalis. Sometimes, considering the patient, you may just need to remove the underlying cause, such as reducing a fever or relieving anxiety.

Atrial Dysrhythmias

ATRIAL TACHYCARDIA

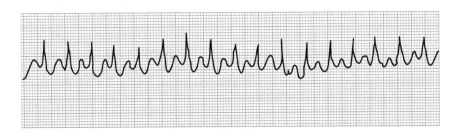

Figure 2-3. Atrial Tachycardia

Definition: Notice this dysrhythmia is no longer called sinus; it is called ATRIAL tachycardia. This should be a clue to you that the source of impulse is no longer coming from the SA node. As mentioned earlier, the SA node usually can only fire up to 150 beats per minute, so as you will see, the rate in atrial tachycardia is faster than this. What has happened in atrial tachycardia is that an ectopic focus in the atria has taken over the pacemaking function of the heart. Atrial tachycardia is always over 150 beats per minute. It is extremely dangerous because cardiac output will almost always be compromised. Also, this dysrhythmia indicates that some type of pathology may be present for an ectopic area to be involved in the first place! However, extreme stress, anxiety, or even digitalis toxicity can cause this dysrhythmia. It also may be idiopathic.

📋 Interpreting the Strip

Step 1: Scan the strip: P waves, QRS complexes, and T waves will always be present, BUT you may not always see the Ps and the Ts. The faster the rate is, the fewer P waves and T waves you will see. These will be hidden within the QRS complexes. However, you know T waves must be present or ventricles could not contract again, since they must repolarize—and this is what T waves represent! The strip will look consistent with no abnormal or premature waveforms. You will notice that the strip appears very "busy." There will not many spaces between the QRS waveforms because of the fast rate.

Step 2: Rates: The ventricular rate is 170, and the atrial rate is 170. Again, sometimes you have to guess at the atrial rate since you may not be sure if you're seeing P waves or T waves. However, the rate is the clue. With atrial tachycardia, the ventricular rate will be over 150 beats per minute, because remember the SA node cannot pace above 150. In atrial tach, the atrial rates and the ventricular rates are the same, so you can make a pretty good assumption from this information.

Step 3: Conduction ratio: 1:1. As mentioned above, the atrial rate and the ventricular rate will be the same. The atrial contractions and the ventricular contractions are "related." As explained above, you sometimes have to take this on good faith, knowing the dysrhythmia is atrial tachycardia.

Step 4: Rhythm: The rhythm for atrial tachycardia usually will be regular. Sometimes you can only "march" the Rs since you cannot see the Ps. However, by knowing the pathophysiology of atrial tach, you can make the assumption that the Ps to Ps would be regular if not hidden.

Step 5: PR interval: This will usually be normal (0.12 to 0.20 seconds) or unable to be obtained because of the fast rate.

Step 6: QRS complex: This will be with normal limits (0.12 seconds or less). This is a very important part in determining if the rhythm is atrial tachycardia. For the rhythm to be this, the QRS complex MUST be normal. You will hear this sometimes called a narrow QRS. You will learn later on that if the rate is fast and you cannot see P waves and the QRS is widened (more than 0.12 seconds), the dysrhythmia is something else—something very dangerous! Therefore, in determining atrial tachycardia, you need to look not only at the rate, but also the width of the QRS complex! THIS IS MOST IMPORTANT!

Step 7: Identify the dysrhythmia: Atrial tachycardia.

Step 8: Determine the source of impulse: Atria.

Interventions/Treatments

The heart definitely needs to be slowed down. No one can tolerate this rate for an extended period of time. Think about the stress this is putting on even a healthy heart. The heart is having to work much harder and is requiring more and more oxygen, and cardiac output is compromised because the ventricles do not have time to fill. The heart is working overtime but with less efficiency. To slow the heart down, beta blockers or calcium channel blockers could be used. Vagal stimulation is something that can be used in an emergency. A newer drug that is being used is amiodarone. A drug that is used specifically for this dysrhythmia is adenosine. Synchronized cardioversion is also an option.

Extra tip: Sometimes you may hear the term *supraventricular tachycardia*. This term really means any type of tachycardia that is occurring above the ventricles and being initiated outside normal pathways. Atrial tachycardia is the most common of these, and sometimes you will hear *atrial tachycardia* and *supraventricular tachycardia* used interchangeably.

ATRIAL FLUTTER

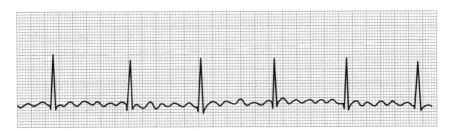

Figure 2-4. Atrial Flutter

Definition: Once again an ectopic focus in the atria is pacing the heart. However, now it is firing the atria at a much faster rate than the focus causing atrial tachycardia was. In fact, it is firing the atria so rapidly that the ventricles cannot possibly respond that fast. The AV node recognizes this and starts to protect the ventricles. It does this by letting a certain number of impulses through the AV node. Therefore, in atrial flutter, the **atrial rate** will be in the range of 250 to 350 beats per minute! The ventricular rate, however, will be variable, depending on how many impulses get through the AV node. The ventricular rate is usually normal to on the fast side. It would hardly ever be slow. Normal ventricular rate (60 to 100) is referred to as controlled ventricular response, while a ventricular rate of more than 100 beats per minute is referred to as an uncontrolled ventricular response. Usually there is some heart pathology when atrial flutter occurs. It often occurs after recent heart surgery. It is not as common as atrial fibrillation, which will be discussed next.

Interpreting the Strip

Step 1: Scan the strip: P waves, QRS complexes, and T waves will be present. However, there are more P waves than QRS complexes, since the atria are contracting more times than the ventricles. Remember the AV node is protecting the ventricles by not letting all of the impulses through from the atria. You may notice that the P waves have a sawtooth appearance. Sometimes P waves are referred to as F waves or flutter waves. Also, T waves may be hidden, since P waves are occurring so rapidly. How do you know T waves are present? Remember they have to be, otherwise the ventricles could not contract again! This strip will look very "busy" and will look like one you have not seen up to this point.

Step 2: Rates: In the above strip, the ventricular rate is 60, and the atrial rate is 300. This corresponds to the definition given above.

Step 3: Conduction ratio: 5:1. This doesn't always have to be 5:1; it could be conduction ratios such as 4:1, 3:1, and so on.

Step 4: Rhythm: Regular with conduction ratio. Atrial and ventricular rhythm will be regular as long as the conduction ratio is the same.

Step 5: PR interval: You will be unable to determine this, because which P waves would you count?

Step 6: QRS complex: This will be within normal limits.

Step 7: Identify the dysrhythmia: Atrial flutter.

Step 8: Determine the source of impulse: An ectopic focus in the atria has taken over the pacing of the heart.

 ## Interventions/Treatments

Treatment of atrial flutter is indicated if the ventricular rate is sufficiently rapid to be potentially dangerous for the patient. Classical treatment is digitalization or cardioversion. A beta blocker or calcium channel blocker also can be used to slow the heart rate. This can be followed by an antidysrhythmic medication such as amiodarone.

ATRIAL FIBRILLATION

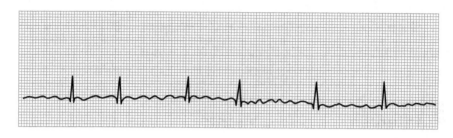

Figure 2-5. Atrial Fibrillation

Definition: Once again an ectopic focus in the atria is pacing the heart. In fact it is believed there may be several spots within the atria firing all at the same time. Again, the AV node comes to the rescue by allowing only certain impulses to reach the ventricles. However, instead of letting a consistent number through like in atrial flutter, it lets impulses through inconsistently. It is thought that perhaps the AV node is bombarded by all the impulses it is receiving. The atria are beating so rapidly that a P wave will not be seen. Instead, a "nervous baseline" will appear before QRS complexes. Something you should notice very quickly is that the ventricles will NOT have a regular rhythm. The causes for atrial fibrillation are numerous and can include conditions such as abnormal heart values, coronary artery disease, hypertension, and electrolyte imbalances.

Interpreting the Strip

Step 1: Scan the strip: You will not be able to identify P waves and probably also not T waves, since they will be hidden by all the activity occurring within the atria. QRS complexes will be present.

Step 2: Rates: The ventricular rate is 60, and you will not be able to determine the atrial rate since you cannot see P waves. (The ventricular rate can be normal or on the fast side, depending on how many impulses are getting through the AV node.)

Step 3: Conduction ratio: You will not be able to determine this.

Step 4: Rhythm: You will not be able to determine the atrial rhythm, but the ventricular rhythm will be **IRREGULAR.**

Step 5: PR interval: You will not be able to determine this.

Step 6: QRS complex: This is normal.

Step 7: Identify the dysrhythmia: Atrial fibrillation.

Step 8: Determine the source of impulse: The source of impulse is from ectopic foci in the atria.

Interventions/Treatments

Treatment of atrial fibrillation is indicated if the ventricular rate is sufficiently rapid to be potentially dangerous to the patient. Classical treatment is digitalization or cardioversion. Beta blockers or calcium channel blockers are other options. Sometimes if the ventricular rate is not dangerously high, the patient may schedule an elective procedure of cardioversion to alleviate the dysrhythmia. Also, a procedure known as ablation therapy may be performed; this involves locating the ectopic foci and destroying them. (TIP: Atrial fibrillation is a common dysrhythmia, especially as individuals age. It can lead to thrombus formation and therefore can put an individual at risk for a cerebral vascular accident. Therefore, anticoagulant therapy is usually indicated in the presence of atrial fibrillation.)

Before your next break, let's test how much you have learned. Fill in the blanks on each cardiac strip and then interpret the dysrhythmia. Good luck!

QUIZ # 4

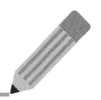

1.

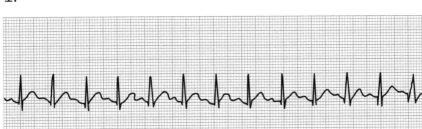

Figure 2-6.

A. P waves, QRS complexes, and T waves present? _____

B. Rate: Ventricular _____ Atrial _____

C. Conduction ratio: _____

D. Rhythm: Ventricular _____ Atrial _____

E.   PR interval: _____

F.   QRS complex: _____

G.   Interpretation: _____

H.   Source of impulse: _____

2.

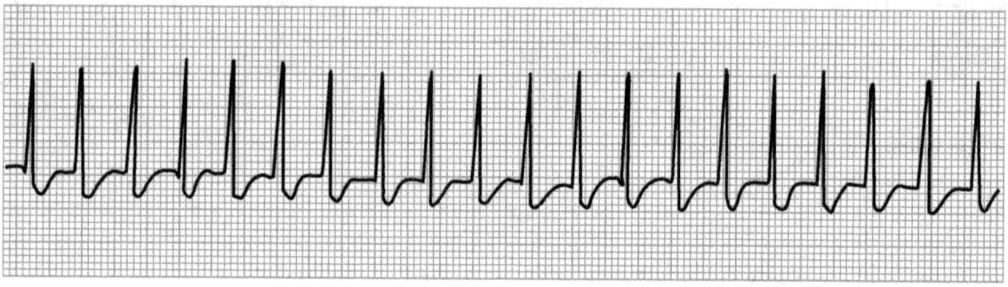

Figure 2-7.

A.   P waves, QRS complexes, and T waves
     present? _____

B.   Rate: Ventricular _____ Atrial _____

C.   Conduction ratio: _____

D. Rhythm: Ventricular _____ Atrial _____

E. PR interval: _____

F. QRS complex: _____

G. Interpretation: _____

H. Source of impulse: _____

Continue reading for the correct answers!

QUIZ # 4 ANSWERS

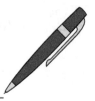

1. A. P waves, QRS complexes, and T waves present? Yes

   B. Rate: Ventricular: 130   Atrial 130

   C. Conduction ratio: 1:1

   D. Rhythm: Ventricular: Regular   Atrial: Regular

   E. PR interval: Normal

   F. QRS complex: Normal

   G. Interpretation: Sinus tachycardia

   H. Source of impulse: SA Node

2. A. P waves, QRS complexes, and T waves present? No, can only see QRS complexes.

   B. Rate: Ventricular: 200 Atrial: unable to determine (on faith—see below)

C. Conduction ratio: 1:1 (on faith—see below)

D. Rhythm: Ventricular: Regular   Atrial: Regular (on faith—see below)

E. PR interval: Unable to determine

F. QRS complex: Normal (This is important!)

G. Interpretation: Considering the ventricular rate and the regular rhythm and the normal (narrow) QRS complex, you should interpret this as atrial tachycardia. Then you could say that the atrial activity is hidden because of the fast rate. Atrial rate, you would know then, would be 200, and the conduction ratio would be 1:1. Source of impulse is an ectopic area in the atria. As indicated above, you have to take some of this "on faith" after interpreting the dysrhythmia.

Well, how did you do?

Take a break!

Reward yourself! You are on your way to becoming a GREAT cardiac nurse!

BREAK!

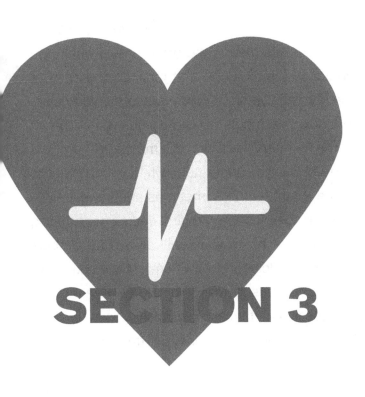

SECTION 3

Atrioventricular Blocks

FIRST-DEGREE BLOCK

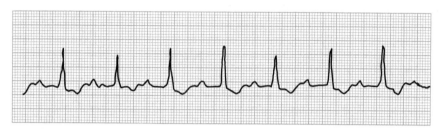

Figure 3-1. First-Degree Heart Block

Definition: A first-degree block is one of the types of blocks known as an AV block. This means the problem lies within the AV node. Remember this is the node that receives the impulse from the SA node normally before it continues to the ventricles. In a first-degree block, the impulse is simply delayed in the AV node. Therefore, the PR interval will be more than 0.20 seconds! That's all there is to it! Can you understand why it is important to always measure the PR interval? (Sometimes another dysrhythmia may be present in combination with first-degree heart block, but since this is a basics book, yours will always be a sinus rhythm except for the first-degree block.) Some of the causes of this dysrhythmia are as follows: diseases of the AV node, electrolyte imbalances, myocardial infarction, and medications such as digitalis. This dysrhythmia also can occur in well-trained athletes.

Interpreting the Strip

Step 1: Scan the strip: P waves, QRS complexes, and T waves will all be present and normal.

Step 2: Rates: Ventricular rate is 70; atrial rate is 70. These are both normal.

Step 3: Conduction ratio: 1:1. For every atrial contraction, there is a ventricular contraction. The impulse is just delayed in the AV node, as denoted by a longer PR interval.

Step 4: Rhythm: Regular.

Step 5: PR Interval: **PROLONGED! It is more than the normal 0.12 to 0.20 seconds or 3 to 5 tiny blocks on the EKG strip. This is the clue to this dysrhythmia!**

Step 6: QRS complex: Within normal limits—0.12 seconds or less.

Step 7: Identify the dysrhythmia: Since the only abnormality is an extended PR interval, the interpretation should be first-degree AV block.

Step 8: Determine the source of impulse: SA node. With this dysrhythmia, the impulse is still coming from the SA node; it just is being delayed in the AV node.

Interventions/Treatments

Usually with this type of block, no treatment is indicated. You should just watch it to make sure it does not progress into a second-degree AV block. These types of blocks are discussed next.

Second-Degree Blocks

Second-degree blocks are not as simple as first-degree blocks. To begin with, there are two types of second-degree blocks.

The two types of second-degree blocks are as follows:

1. Mobitz I or type I (Wenckebach)

2. Mobitz II or type II (classical)

With a first-degree block, all of the impulses from the SA node reached the ventricles; they only were delayed. However, with a second-degree block (both types), some of the impulses from the SA node are **blocked** at the AV node. Each type of second-degree block will be discussed next.

MOBITZ I OR TYPE I (WENCKEBACH)

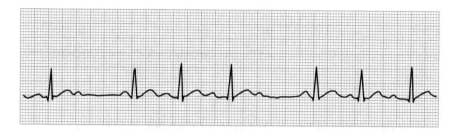

Figure 3-2. Mobitz I, Type 1, Wenckebach Second-Degree Heart Block

Definition: With this block, the AV node is still the problem. The AV node requires a progressively longer interval of time to transmit an impulse, and finally an impulse fails to be conducted to the ventricles. When the next impulse arrives, the rested AV node is able to transmit the impulse in a normal time, but the next one requires a longer time, and the cycle continues. Some of the causes for this dysrhythmia include diseases of the AV node, myocardial infarction, post cardiac surgery, myocarditis, and medications such as digitalis, beta blockers, and calcium channel blockers. This dysrhythmia also can occur in well-trained athletes.

 ## Interpreting the Strip

Step 1: Scan the strip: P waves, QRS complexes, and T waves are all present, but there are more P waves than QRS complexes.

Step 2: Rates: The ventricular rate is 70, and the atrial rate is 90. The ventricular rate is lower because some of the impulses are not conducted.

Step 3: Conduction ratio: 1:1 ,then 1:0, then the cycle starts again.

Step 4: Rhythm: The ventricular rhythm (Rs to Rs) will be irregular since the PR intervals are getting progressively longer and some QRS complexes are dropped. However, if you march the atrial rhythm (Ps to Ps), you will see that rhythm is regular.

Step 5: PR interval: It starts out normal (0.12 to 0.20 seconds) but gets progressively longer with each impulse (more than 0.20 seconds) until one entire impulse is completely blocked!

Step 6: QRS complex: This will be within normal limits.

Step 7: Identify the dysrhythmia: Mobitz I or type I (Wenckebach). It always is important to look at PR intervals (each PR interval), or you may misinterpret this one. Observing that the PR interval is becoming progressively longer until one is dropped is the clue to realizing that this is Mobitz I or type I or Wenckebach (all the same) second-degree AV block.

Step 8: Determine the source of impulse: It is still the SA node; the impulse is just being delayed and ultimately blocked in the AV node!

Interventions/Treatments

Usually no symptoms are present, and no treatment is necessary. If the ventricular rate is slow and the patient is showing signs and symptoms of decreased cardiac output, atropine may be given. The need for a pacemaker is rare. Usually this dysrhythmia is temporary. However, you should watch and make sure this dysrhythmia does not progress into the other type of second-degree block, which will be discussed next.

MOBITZ II OR TYPE II (CLASSICAL)

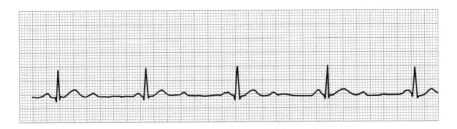

Figure 3-3. Mobitz II, Type 2, Classical Second-Degree Heart Block

Definition: This dysrhythmia is a more serious one than Mobitz I. With this dysrhythmia, only a certain ratio of impulses that reach the AV node are transmitted, and the rest are blocked. Since the rate of the impulses coming from the atria is usually normal, can you imagine what this would do to the ventricular rate if some of them are blocked and cannot get through to the ventricles? You are correct! You generally will see a SLOW ventricular rate with this type of block, and this can be a problem. Why? You are correct again! Cardiac output will be affected and can very well be decreased. Do you remember which part of the heart is mainly responsible for cardiac output? The ventricles are, of course! The cause of this dysrhythmia is usually related to pathology of the conduction system, which can be caused by things such as myocardial infarction, post cardiac surgery, heart failure, and medications such as digitalis.

📋 Interpreting the Strip

Step 1: Scan the strip: P waves, QRS complexes, and T waves are all present, but there are more P waves than QRS complexes. Also, sometimes with this dysrhythmia, the T waves may be hidden, or it may be hard to tell the difference between P waves and T waves. (Hint: To tell the difference, locate a P wave and measure the distance to the next P wave. They should all be the same distance apart. In other words, the rhythm for P to P will be regular, and they will "march." This is how you can tell a P wave from a T wave with this dysrhythmia.

Step 2: Rates: The ventricular rate is 50, and the atrial rate is 90. Notice the atrial rate is greater than the ventricular rate because of the blocked impulses.

Step 3: Conduction ratio: This can vary in this type of block. It will never be 1:1. It can be 2:1, 3:1, 4:1, and so on. In the dysrhythmia in Figure 3.3, it is 2:1.

Step 4: Rhythm: The atrial rhythm (P to P) is regular. The ventricular rhythm (R to R) is regular. The rhythm for this type of dysrhythmia will always be regular as long as the conduction ratio is consistent and the same. If the conduction ratio were to change, the rhythm would be irregular.

Step 5: PR interval: In the above dysrhythmia and with Mobitz II in general, the PR interval cannot be determined. Which P wave would you measure?

Step 6: QRS complex: The QRS complex will be within normal limits (0.12 seconds or less).

Step 7: Identify the dysrhythmia: Mobitz II or type II or classical AV second-degree heart block. (These are all the same; this dysrhythmia can be called Mobitz II, type II, or classical second-degree heart block).

Step 8: Determine the source of impulse: SA node. A certain ratio of the impulses is being blocked in the AV node.

Treatments/Interventions

As stated above, this is a more serious type of heart block. Why? The problem lies within the AV node. The SA node will be firing at a normal rate of 60 to 100 beats per minute. Therefore, the atrial rate will be within normal limits. Remember some of these impulses will be "blocked" in the AV node. What if the conduction ratio is 2:1? That means for every atrial contraction, only one is reaching the ventricles and causing them to contract. What if the conduction ratio is 3:1? That means for every atrial contraction, only every third one is reaching the ventricles and causing them to contract. Therefore, can you see how a conduction ratio of 2:1 is the best you can have if the dysrhythmia is Mobitz II? What if the atrial rate is 100 beats per minute, which is the best it can be and still be normal? What if the conduction ratio is 2:1, which is the best it can be? In this example, the ventricular rate would be 50 beats per minute, which is slow and which could affect cardiac output. Are you getting the picture? What if the atrial rate was 60 (which is still normal) and the conduction ratio was 3:1? What would the ventricular rate be with this dysrhythmia? You're correct again. It would be 20 beats per minute, and cardiac output certainly would be affected!

Therefore, the cardiac output must always be assessed with this dysrhythmia. A pacemaker may be indicated. Also, this dysrhythmia can quickly progress into a third-degree block, where a pacemaker definitely will be indicated.

Review

Before you continue with the AV blocks, take a quiz to make sure you are retaining all of this information. Set your watch to go and good luck!

QUIZ # 5

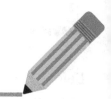

Match the following:

1. All impulses from the
   SA node are conducted
   through the AV node; they
   are just delayed.

   __A. Mobitz I, type 1
   (Wenckebach)

2. With this block only a
   certain ratio of impulses
   reaches the ventricles; the
   rest are blocked.

   __B. First-degree block

3. With this block, impulses
   are delayed progressively
   longer until one is finally
   blocked completely, and
   then the cycle starts over
   again.

   __C. Mobitz II, type 2 (classical)

   Continue reading for the correct answers!

QUIZ # 5 ANSWERS

1. B

2. C

3. A

How did you do?

If you answered all correctly, take a break and reward yourself!

We don't want to have brain overload at this point!

If you did not answer all correctly, go back and review for a few more minutes.

Welcome back! Now you need to learn about the last of the AV blocks.

THIRD-DEGREE HEART BLOCK

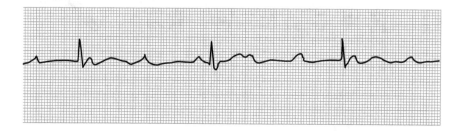

Figure 3-4. Third-Degree Heart Block

Definition: Third-degree heart block is also called a complete heart block. This block is just as its name indicates. All of the impulses from the SA node are blocked completely so that none of the impulses get through to the ventricles.

One question you might have is, how are the ventricles contracting if all impulses are being blocked?

Remember that at the beginning of this book, you were told that if the SA node and the AV node failed to initiate an impulse, the ventricles would take over. This is exactly what happens with a third-degree heart block. The ventricles are being paced by the ventricles themselves. The atria are being paced by a higher center, probably the SA node. Since the impulses coming from the atria are being blocked at the AV node, the ventricles must take over, or no cardiac output!

BUT, you must remember that the ventricles pace very slowly, and usually they cannot keep this up for a long period of time. Therefore, this is a very dangerous dysrhythmia! Think about how cardiac output is being compromised. Remember how the ideal situation is for all parts of the heart to work together. That is, normally the atria fill with blood, and then the ventricles fill with this blood. With third-degree heart block, these parts of the heart are working independently. The causes for this type of dysrhythmia are numerous. Certainly all of the causes for the previous types of blocks can lead to a complete heart block. Definitely there is pathology of the AV node that can be caused by, in addition to the cardiac situations already discussed, toxins, hypoxia, and hypothyroidism.

 ## Interpreting the Strip

Step 1: Scan the strip: P waves, QRS complexes, and T waves all seem to be present. However, you should notice something "strange" about this strip. The P waves do not seem to occur where they normally should in relation to the QRS complexes. Remember, however, the atria are contracting independently, and the ventricles are contracting independently! (Hint: In the clinical setting, we sometimes refer to the Ps and QRS complexes being divorced and no longer married.)

Step 2: Rates: The ventricular rate is 30, and the atrial rate is 80. Notice that they are different. With a third-degree heart block, the ventricular rate will most likely be toward the slow side since this is the nature of the ventricles. The atrial rate will usually be normal (60 to 100 beats per minute) since they are being fired by the SA node. Remember the SA node is firing normally; the impulses are just being blocked in the AV node.

Step 3: Conduction ratio: 0:0. No impulses are being conducted from the atria to the ventricles.

Step 4: Rhythm: The atrial rhythm will be regular. The Ps to Ps will "march." The Rs to Rs will be regular, and they will "march." (Hint: This is how you will be able to tell a P wave from a T wave).

Step 5: PR interval: Cannot determine.

Step 6: QRS complex: Normal to widened. Remember the ventricles are pacing themselves. Therefore, if a spot high up in the ventricles is pacing, the QRS complex may be normal (0.12 seconds or less). However, if a spot lower in the ventricles is pacing, the QRS complex will be widened (more than 0.12 seconds or more than 3 tiny blocks on the EKG paper).

Step 7: Identify the dysrhythmia: Third-degree heart block, which is also called complete heart block

Step 8: Determine the source of impulse: The source of impulse for the atria is the SA node; the source of impulse for the ventricles is the ventricles themselves!

 Treatments/Interventions

This dysrhythmia is an emergency and requires a pacemaker. Cardiac output is seriously compromised.

Ventricular Dysrhythmias

You are **ALMOST** finished with all the information you need to know to have a basic understanding of interpreting cardiac dysrhythmias. However, you do have one last group of dysrhythmias to review: ventricular dysrhythmias. These are very important, because they can lead to life-threatening situations. So as a nurse, you must be able to recognize these and to respond quickly!

Just as the name denotes, these dysrhythmias arise from the ventricles. Since the impulse is originating in an ectopic area of the ventricles, the QRS complex will be wide and "different looking."

You are going to learn about the basic ventricular dysrhythmias. They are as follows: premature ventricular contractions, ventricular tachycardia, and ventricular fibrillation.

Let's get you started!

PREMATURE VENTRICULAR CONTRACTIONS

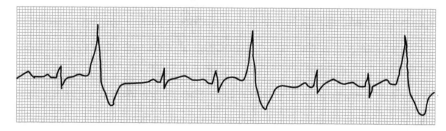

Figure 3-5. Premature Ventricular Contractions (PVCs)

Definition: A premature ventricular contraction (PVC) is a contraction of the ventricles that is initiated by the ventricles. Therefore, there is no P wave before the QRS complex, since the atria are not contracting. A PVC comes too quickly in the underlying rhythm, so it is termed "premature." Some of the main characteristics of PVCs are as follows:

1. They occur early in the cycle.

2. They are not preceded by a P wave.

3. They have a wide and bizarre QRS complex.

4. They have a T wave opposite in direction to that of the QRS complex.

5. They are usually followed by a full compensatory pause. What this means is that the next normal contraction after a PVC is stopped while the ventricles depolarize. However, the rhythm continues on schedule with the next contraction.

6. PVCs can be classified in several ways. One is by using a system to describe their originating site. They can be classified as being unifocal or multifocal.

   Unifocal PVCs originate from the same site in the ventricles. How will you be able to tell this? The answer is: The PVCs will all look alike! It is that simple.

   Multifocal PVCs, on the other hand, originate from different sites in the ventricles. How do you suppose they will look? You are correct! They will look different from each other.

   PVCs also can be classified as to how often they are occurring, or as to what pattern they are exhibiting. *Bigeminy* and *trigeminy* are terms that are used in this classification system. With bigeminy every other ventricular contraction is a PVC, whereas with trigeminy every third ventricular contraction is a PVC. PVCs can also be classified as couplets, which means two PVCs are occurring together in a row.

   The causes for PVCs are varied and sometimes unclear. Some possible causes are underlying heart disease, hypertension, chemical imbalances, certain medications, alcohol, anxiety, and caffeine.

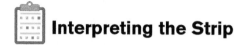

Interpreting the Strip

Step 1: Scan the strip: P waves, QRS complexes, and T waves are present for the underlying rhythm. Notice the big unusual complexes; circle these; these are PVCs. Notice there are no P waves preceding the PVCs.

Step 2: Rates: The ventricular rate is 50, and the atrial rate is 50. Notice we do not count a PVC as a ventricular contraction, because it gives very little cardiac output. Why? The PVC has occurred early, so the ventricles have not had adequate time to fill with blood.

Step 3: Conduction ratio: 0:0 for PVCs. There is no atrial conduction/contraction preceding the PVC.

Step 4: Rhythm: Usually full compensatory pause following the PVC, and then the underlying rhythm continues.

Step 5: PR interval: Unable to determine since no atrial contraction (P wave) precedes PVC.

Step 6: QRS complex: Widened—more than 0.12 seconds for the PVCs.

Step 7: Identify the dysrhythmia: 3 unifocal PVCs.

Step 8: Determine the source of impulse: Origin of impulse for the PVCs is from the ventricles. There will be a different origin of impulse for the underlying rhythm.

Interventions/Treatments

PVCs will usually only be treated if cardiac output is being compromised. Usually this will be more of a possibility with large numbers of PVCs or patterns such as bigeminy. Multifocal PVCs also indicate more irritability within the myocardium. If cardiac output is being compromised, lidocaine has been the drug of choice for many years. However, two other drugs being used now are amiodarone and procainamide.

VENTRICULAR TACHYCARDIA

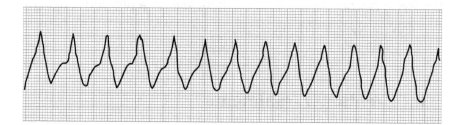

Figure 3-6. Ventricular Tachycardia

Definition: Ventricular tachycardia (v-tach) is defined as a series of multiple (three or more) PVCs occurring in a row, usually at a rate of 100 beats per minute or more. (Hint: What do we call this v-tach? Remember, normally if the ventricles initiate an impulse, they do so in an emergency situation, and they pace slowly. With v-tach, they are irritable/ischemic, so they pace very fast.)

Answer a question at this time. What do you think is happening to cardiac output during ventricular tachycardia?

You are correct once again! There's not much cardiac output at all with v-tach. This is an emergency situation!

However, there's one more piece of information you need regarding ventricular tachycardia. This dysrhythmia can be classified as "v-tach with a pulse" or "v-tach without a pulse." Of course, you have to observe and assess the client to be able to determine this. If the client has a pulse and is conscious, this is a better situation than v-tach without a pulse (neither are very good, however).

If the latter is occurring, the client is treated the same as one with ventricular fibrillation. This dysrhythmia is discussed next.

Even if the client is displaying ventricular tachycardia on the monitor and is conscious with a pulse, the health-care provider has to act quickly because the ventricles cannot continue to pace for a long period of time. Also, remember that ventricular tachycardia is basically many PVCs in a row, and there is little cardiac output from PVCs.

Answer another question at this time. With v-tach, what part of the heart has taken over the complete pacing of the heart?

You are correct again! The ventricles have, because remember what v-tach is. It is a rhythm of all PVCs, and with the dysrhythmia of v-tach, it is completely PVCs—nothing else—no underlying rhythm to help out. That's why this dysrhythmia is such an emergency!

Another problem with v-tach is that it can very quickly change to ventricular fibrillation!

Ventricular tachycardia is associated with irritability of the ventricles. The cause can be related to a complication associated with a myocardial infarction such as ischemia. Cardiomyopathy can be another cause. Structural heart disorders may be a cause, as well as a disorder called the long QT syndrome. Metabolic and electrolyte disturbances may also be involved in the development of this dysrhythmia.

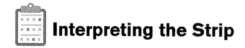 **Interpreting the Strip**

Step 1: Scan the strip: P waves, QRS complexes, and T waves are not present. Only widened and bizarre QRS complexes are present.

Step 2: Rates: The ventricular rate is 140, and the atrial rate is 0. Notice we have to count the multiple PVCs here because that is what ventricular tachycardia is and that is all we have!

Step 3: Conduction ratio: 0:0.

Step 4: Rhythm: Regular, although sometimes v-tach can be slightly irregular.

Step 5: PR interval: None.

Step 6: QRS complex: Widened—more than 0.12 seconds (This is important!)

Step 7: Identify the dysrhythmia: Ventricular tachycardia.

Step 8: Determine the source of impulse: Ventricles.

Interventions/Treatments

For v-tach with a pulse present: Cardioversion, followed by amio-darone, procainamide, or lidocaine.

For v-tach without a pulse: Treat as ventricular fibrillation (see next dysrhythmia).

An implanted cardioverter/defibrillator could be an option for persistent problems.

VENTRICULAR FIBRILLATION

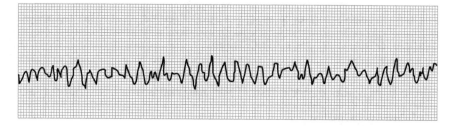

Figure 3-7. Ventricular Fibrillation

Definition: With *ventricular fibrillation* (v-fib), numerous ectopic foci in the ventricles are firing simultaneously. There is no effective contraction of the heart, and the client will have no pulse. If this dysrhythmia is not terminated, the client will die within minutes.

Fortunately, v-fib is one of the easiest dysrhythmias to recognize. The only other possible thing it can be is electrical interference or a disconnected electrode. If your client talks to you when you go to check on him or her, it is NOT v-fib!

The causes of v-fib are numerous. Many times this dysrhythmia occurs as a result of a myocardial infarction. Other possible causes are cardiomyopathies, post cardiac surgery, and electrocution accidents.

 Interpreting the Strip

Step 1: Scan the strip: P waves, QRS complexes, and T waves are not present. This dysrhythmia presents as a wavy baseline.

Step 2: Rates: The ventricular and the atrial rate are both zero. There is no cardiac output.

Step 3: Conduction ratio: 0:0.

Step 4: Rhythm: None.

Step 5: PR interval: None.

Step 6: QRS complex: None.

Step 7: Identify the dysrhythmia: Ventricular fibrillation.

Step 8: Determine the source of impulse: Ventricles.

Interventions/Treatments

Defibrillation is the only treatment. Cardiopulmonary resuscitation (CPR) is necessary until defibrillation is successful or terminated. Drugs such as epinephrine, amiodarone, lidocaine, magnesium, and procainamide may be given.

YOU ARE FINISHED—ALMOST!

There's two more dysrhythmias that you should learn. Continue reading to learn about the first one!

Asystole

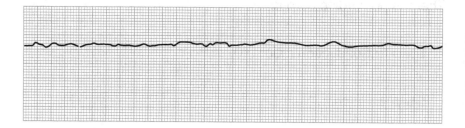

Figure 3-8. Asystole

As you can see in Figure 3-8, there is no electrical activity occurring within the heart with this dysrhythmia. The treatment for this dysrhythmia is CPR. Sometimes in the emergency room, clients may be given electrolytes or epinephrine to try to alleviate this dysrhythmia.

Again, the causes are numerous. Some of them are as follows: myocardial infarction, hypothermia, drowning, smoke inhalation, massive bleeding with resulting hypotension, hyperkalemia, and drug overdose.

Pulseless Electrical Activity

With this condition, the patient is displaying a rhythm on the cardiac monitor in which the patient should have a pulse. However, upon assessing the person, there is no pulse—the patient is having a cardiac arrest! This condition is beyond the scope of this book, but you should be aware that it exists. There are certain conditions that are associated with this disorder. These are known as the Hs and the Ts because the causative conditions either begin with an H or a T. After you have mastered this beginning book, research this condition and be familiar with some of the causes. As a beginning clinician, just be aware that technology can never replace the assessment skills of the nurse. Always assess your patient and make sure what the monitor is telling you matches what you see with your patient.

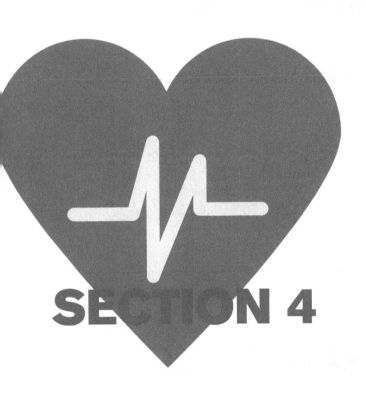

SECTION 4

Practice Strips

The author has divided your practice strips into sections to help you know where to begin. These sections are as follows: sinoatrial dysrhythmias, AV blocks, and ventricular dysrhythmias. At the end, all of the dysrhythmias are combined to really test how efficient you have become!

The answers to all are found on the very last page of this book. Remember to use your step-by-step guide as you attempt to interpret the dysrhythmias. Do your best!

SINOATRIAL DYSRHYTHMIAS (SECTION II)

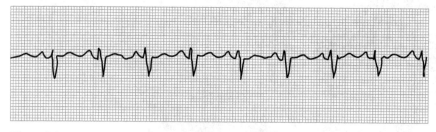

Figure 4-1.

Interpretation: _____

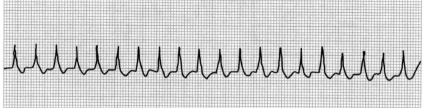

Figure 4-2.

Interpretation: _____

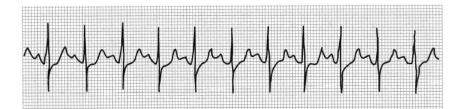

Figure 4-3.

Interpretation: _____

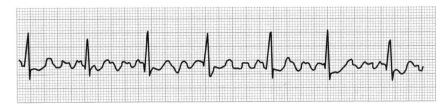

Figure 4-4.

Interpretation: _____

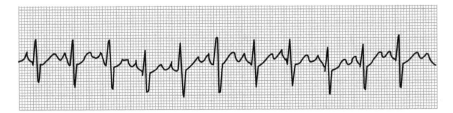

Figure 4-5.

Interpretation: _____

Answers are on the last page.

How did you do?

If you are having trouble, go back and review the pages on sinus and atrial dysrhythmias. If you had no trouble with this, continue!

ATRIOVENTRICULAR BLOCKS (SECTION III)

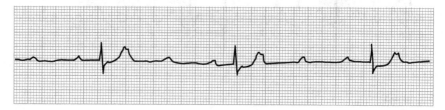

Figure 4-6.

Interpretation: _____

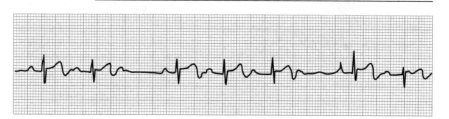

Figure 4-7.

Interpretation: _____

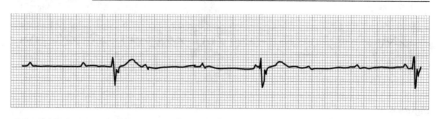

Figure 4-8.

Interpretation: _____

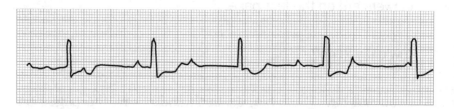

Figure 4-9.

Interpretation: _____

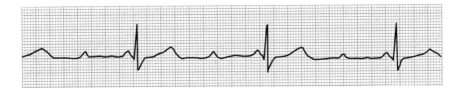

Figure 4-10.

Interpretation: _____

VENTRICULAR DYSRHYTHMIAS (SECTION III)

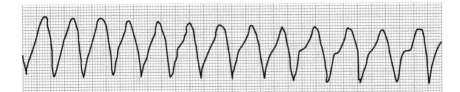

Figure 4-11.

Interpretation: _____

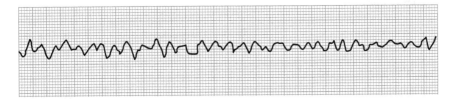

Figure 4-12.

Interpretation: _____

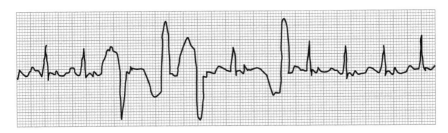

Figure 4-13.

Interpretation: _____

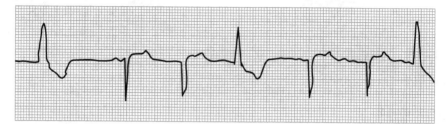

Figure 4-14.

Interpretation: _____

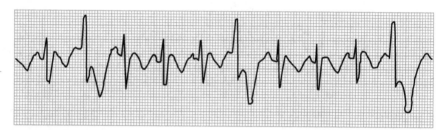

Figure 4-15.

Interpretation: _____

ALL DYSRHYTHMIAS

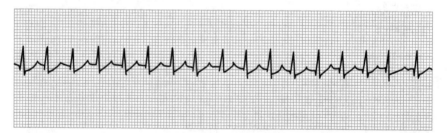

Figure 4-16.

Interpretation: _____

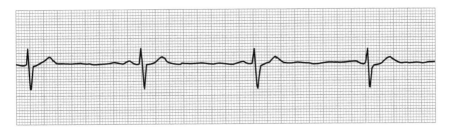

Figure 4-17.

Interpretation: _____

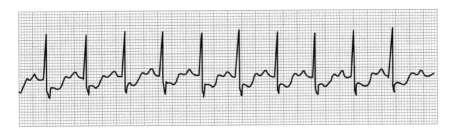

Figure 4-18.

Interpretation: _____

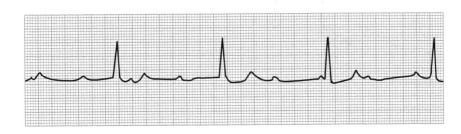

Figure 4-19.

Interpretation: _____

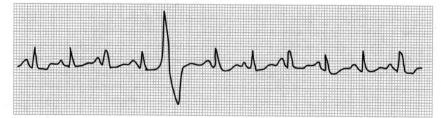

Figure 4–20.

Interpretation: _____

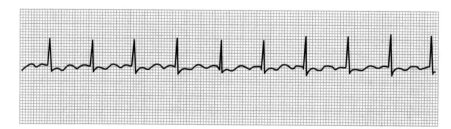

Figure 4-21.

Interpretation: _____

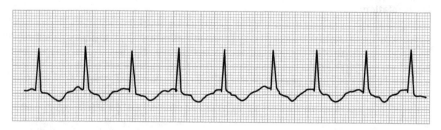

Figure 4-22.

Interpretation: _____

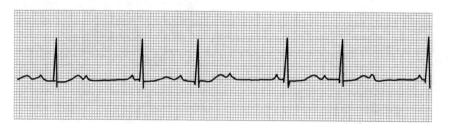

Figure 4-23.

Interpretation: _____

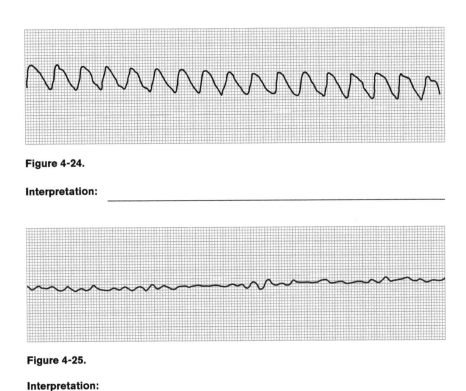

Figure 4-24.

Interpretation: _____

Figure 4-25.

Interpretation: _____

All of the answers are listed next. Check and see how you have done! You are truly on your way to becoming a GREAT cardiac nurse. Go celebrate! You have worked hard!

Answers to Section IV Strips

SINOATRIAL DYSRHYTHMIAS

4.1. Normal sinus rhythm

4.2. Atrial tachycardia

4.3. Sinus tachycardia

4.4. Atrial flutter

4.5. Sinus tachycardia

AV BLOCKS

4.6. Second-degree block, Mobitz II, type II, classical

4.7. Second-degree block, Mobitz I, type I, Wenckebach

4.8. Third-degree block

4.9. Third-degree block

4.10. Second-degree block, Mobitz II, type II, classical

VENTRICULAR DYSRHYTHMIAS

4.11. Ventricular tachycardia

4.12. Ventricular fibrillation

4.13. Multifocal premature ventricular contractions

4.14. Trigeminy unifocal premature ventricular contractions

4.15. Quadrigeminy unifocal premature ventricular contractions

ALL DYSRHYTHMIAS

4.16. Atrial tachycardia

4.17. Sinus bradycardia

4.18. Normal Sinus Rhythm - (almost Sinus tachycardia)

4.19. Third-degree block

4.20. Normal sinus rhythm with one premature ventricular contraction (Close to being sinus tachycardia with one premature ventricular contraction)

4.21. Atrial flutter

4.22. Normal sinus rhythm (T wave is just depressed—don't worry—we did not discuss that—you will learn about that later)

4.23. Second-degree block, Mobitz I, type I, Wenckebach

4.24. Ventricular tachycardia

4.25. Ventricular fibrillation

Image Credit

- Copyright © Depositphotos/TopVectors